I0782793

# Re-Organize your diet

# Re-Organize Your Diet
## and improve your lifestyle

### Cristian Ortile

**Translated by Clarissa Cassels**

*"You are free to choose your lifestyle but not the final result"*
**Herbert MacGolfin Shelton**

Reorganize your Diet



This manual offers information and interesting points in general,
regarding health and the correct way of eating. Therefore it
should not be a substitute to doctor's advice, in consideration of
the vast diversity of people interested and the variety of diseases,
and it does not intend to prescribe a diet that can suit anybody.
The publisher and the author accept no responsibility in the case
of  inappropriate use of information.

# Introduction

If we want to improve ourselves the first thing we need to confront is our diet.

Why is this?

First of all a correct diet has a positive impact on our level of physical energy, on our life expectancy, on our mood and our concentration but it is also able to improve the quality of sleep and it has a more efficient effect to prevent (and cure) health issues.

Whatever our objective might be, to start practising a sport, to be more into our job, to have the right determination to reach a certain goal or simply to feel good within ourselves, the first step is to improve what we put into our body, because what we eat ends up becoming part of ourselves and if we eat badly sooner or later we feel unwell.

To eat in a healthy way nowadays has become more complicated than one might think; we can easily go to the supermarket next door and fill up our trolley with all sorts of food dictated by TV adverts that decide what is healthy.

But are these foods really healthy??

We are literally submerged by TV adverts and programs, newspaper articles, blogs and specialized magazines in which we are told what to eat or what not to eat, what makes us lose weight or not, leaving us even more confused.

We end up growing up with the wrong habits and our views of what is right or wrong to eat are just part of teachings and prejudices that we have built up over the years.

Really it's all quite unclear.

Therefore out of curiosity I started to read some books about diet and what at first left me perplexed is the contradictions of the experts among themselves, leaving one confused and not knowing what to cook. Even the most famous scientists had different views so how could I see clearly?

The more I was reading books with opposite views, to my great surprise I realized that their views were not so distant from each other, it was just just that some theories were based more on the positive effects of a type of nourishment while other theories were advising against.

At the beginning the gap between the two ways of thinking seemed wide but the more I analysed the more it was coming closer like water passed through a funnel.

So motivated by the need to clarify myself I did an in-depth research through books, food and diet courses. Finally, from these, I concluded in describing the two most up-to-date and correct diets with advice for daily use, properties of each food and nutrients which are fundamental for us-

This is why this practical booklet was started.

# Summary

# Chapter 1

**What diet to choose?**
**Nutritional value**
**Our body, our car**
**Challenge n°1**

*"The majority of the food we eat is not the result of a choice but of influence"*
**Allen Carr**
(It is easy to control weight if you know how to do it)

# What diet to choose?

The Greek word '*diaitea*', from which the word diet comes from, means lifestyle, therefore a dietary way of life that we human beings follow.
Nowadays, when we talk of diet we think of two to three months, maybe before the summer, in which period of time we follow a short regime with rules on what to eat or not to eat.
Very often the person that decides to lose weight decides on the basis of stories one hears or personal interpretations ending with no results or even worse causing a health risk. Moreover, the advent of the internet has contributed to the publication of many revolutionary diets mainly not scientifically based but only theoretical.

# Nutritional value

When we buy a product we find on the packaging a list of the nutritional values of the food in question.

What are they and what is this for? They are purely theoretical indications but a useful way to understand what we are eating and the positive or negative

| Energy |
| Carbohydrates |
| of which are sugar |
| Fats |
| of which are saturated fatty acids |
| Protein |
| of which is animal protein |
| Fibre |
| Others |

aspects of our diet. To start with we don't have a food composed just of carbohydrates or protein but we have a bit of both in every food. Therefore, the nourishment is considered carbohydrate if it is present in its majority and vice versa, if protein is in prevalence.

In the list below and in the food list under carbohydrates you always see written "of which sugars" and under fats "saturated fatty acids". This is because sugars and saturated fats are part of carbohydrates and fats that we have to watch for and limit their consumption.

When we say "others" we are talking about vitamins and minerals, other very fundamental elements for our health, which are present in small quantities in nearly all food and of fibre, especially present in vegetables to aid the functioning of the bowl.

It is now easy to understand that every food that we consume  has positive and negative aspects to it.

It is not good enough to eat carbohydrates for lunch or proteins in the evening just because we hear it is the way to do it, we must be careful about the type of carbohydrates or proteins we eat.

The quantity of each nutrient varies according to the food, if it is from animal source there will be more proteins but also saturated fats, while vegetables will have more carbohydrates, water and more unsaturated fats (good "fats")

# Our body, our car

Our fuel is carbohydrate.

Anybody who has read any health or dietary book has found this assonance.

All very true and from here we already understand how fundamental carbohydrates are in giving us the energy we need to face the day ahead.

To simplify even further, let us pretend for a moment that our body is really like a car; carbohydrates are, like we said, our fuel, while proteins (the bricks which hold our body) are the luxurious interiors and the smart bodywork, while fats are the seat belts and the tyres and they are there to protect us.

All these elements are fundamental for the car to function and work properly.
No one is part more important than the other, but each must be seen in the right context.
One can have a new and beautiful car, with all the unimaginable security systems, but without fuel the car will not move. If we put in only a little fuel we would need to stop often for fuel. With too much fuel we would feel too heavy and if we introduce the wrong fuel we would need to go to the mechanic.
For this reason carbohydrates are the basis of a healthy diet, which should be 50-60% of what we usually eat. With these proportions the chances of the car breaking down are reduced.
Therefore if we don't take care of our car soon it will start getting ruined, with scratches and bumps, it will get rusty a little at the time and it would be too late to restore it to its original splendour.
To stop that from happening we need very little, a small bit of maintenance each day to keep it beautiful and sparkling and even if years go by the charm remains the same.
This short metaphor is to say that proteins are fundamental but are needed in much smaller quantities than we are made to believe. Each day they should make up 15% of what we eat.

Fats, on the other hand, are our safety systems; driving without safety belts or with worn tyres are a great risk to our health.

Good fats help to protect our body, while bad fats act against the good ones and put us at risk by making us more vulnerable.
They should constitute 30% of our food intake.

After this short lesson in mechanics let us now move on to getting to know these three fundamental nutrients, of which there are positive and negative aspects.


**Challenge °1**

At the end of each chapter we will find this section which presents the challenge to eat well and to carry it through to the end.
They can be taken as a weekly challenge and we can try to follow them throughout the week or as a daily challenge where we try to incorporate one of those meals that we are advised to take.
This first week we read this manual to get some idea of how it works, then from next week onwards we try to carry the weekly challenge on to the end of each chapter.

# Chapter 2

**Carbohydrates (what are they and what do they do?)**
**Complex carbohydrates**
**Gluten**
**Fruit and honey**
**Simple carbohydrates**
**Challenge n°2**

*"We don't know either where our food comes from or where it ends up, we are provisional carriers, distracted consumers and most of the time not aware of it, the ultimate goal is our immediate satisfaction"*
**Paola Maugeri**
(My life at zero impact)

# Carbohydrates

As already seen, whether it is a Mediterranean, oriental or vegetarian diet, a healthy diet is based on carbohydrates which are our the most important source of energy and should constitute 50-60% of what we eat.
During digestion all carbohydrates are broken down and transformed into  glucose, which is simple sugar. This, through hormones like insulin, is carried to the blood and it gives us the energy we need.
The level of sugar in the blood (so called glycaemia) must remain constant to avoid ailments and health issues in the future, for example diabetes.
Carbohydrates can be divided into two types: complex (starch) and simple carbohydrates (sugars).
**Complex carbohydrates release sugars into the blood in a slow and gradual way,** giving us constant energy, meanwhile **simple** carbohydrates have a fast release and **cause our energy levels to fluctuate rapidly, making them go up and down very quickly**, creating a dangerous escalation for our health.

# Complex Carbohydrates

Our diet must be based on complex carbohydrates.
We are talking about **whole wheat cereals**, even
better if in the form of grains, as a whole, so to
maintain their nutritional properties, otherwise lost in
the process of refining.

**Grain,** or **wheat,** that we normally consume as pasta,
bread and pizza, is the main cereal in our diet and it is
an optimum food to be consumed wholemeal because
the refining process that produces white flour
impoverishes the nutritional value of the wheat.
Moreover grain is full of minerals and anti anaemic
agents.
On the other hand, being the most popular, it is also
the most manipulated type of grain, so it is advisable
to insert in the diet varied types of organic and
wholemeal wheat.
There are many types of cereals and it is important to
vary them each day, because there are many different
nutritional values that complement each other giving
our body all the necessary nutrients.
In addition, if we eat the same food every day a form
of addiction is created which causes less nutritional
advantages because our body becomes too
accustomed to it, with the risk of becoming intolerant
in the future (such as with gluten-rich foods).
Every cereal contains optimum nutritional values, is

rich in minerals and vitamins and has good quantities of protein.

**Rice**, also well known, is better as wholemeal, is good for losing weight and is easily digestible, likewise **quinoa**, a cereal with a high protein content and rich in calcium and **millet** which is cleansing and rich in minerals.

**Spelt** is suitable for sporty types as it contains few calories but helps to increase muscle mass and it invigorates muscles, as **oats** do, which are a great strengthener. Also we have **barley** which is refreshing and beneficial to the nervous system, and then there is **rye** which stimulates the metabolism and is energising. **Amaranth**, good for the heart and liver, **buckwheat** (that, in spite of the name, is not actually a grain but for its characteristics is associated as one) is warming and mineralising.

Last but not least we have **kamut**, which is an ancestor of wheat, and **maize,** another well-known cereal, with relaxing properties that is used mainly to make polenta flour or sweets, and to make **gluten-free pasta**, as rice, millet, amaranth, quinoa and buckwheat can also do.

Recent developments have also shown that also oats are to be considered gluten-free although up to not long it was considered to be a cereal containing some gluten likely due to the fact that when it was cultivated it became contaminated with wheat, rye and spelt

# Dehusked or pearled grain?

Pearled grain goes through a kind of process of refinery that takes away the outermost coat, while the ones that are de-husked are simply picked as they come, and so they are to be preferred to pearled grain. If however we consume food coming from farms that use chemical fertilizers (to be avoided in any case!) it is better to favour the pearled grain as most of the chemical residue is found on the external husk. Another advantage of pearled grain is that it does not require soaking as other types of cereals do.

# Gluten

The graph shows the average amount of gluten content of various cereals. Wheat contains the greatest quantity. Gluten is the wheat

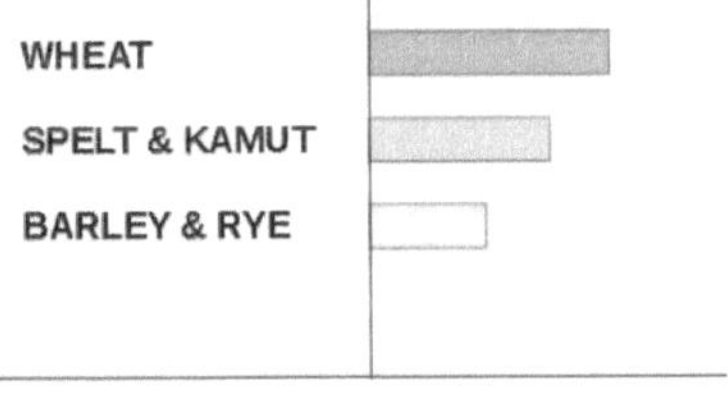


protein. The name comes from gluten which means 'glue' and it is the gluey part of the grain, the part that with a bit of water holds the flour together during the preparation of bread and pizza.

Some cereals without gluten might state on the package "May contain gluten" due to the fact that it is produced industrially in a factory where other types of cereal are also produced and runs the risk of coming into contact with other grains or flours that do contain gluten, for example a production line that works on other cereals.
For those who are intolerant even to the tiniest contact, this can bring about nasty side effects such as cramps and intestinal pains.
Then there are those who are not so sensitive to the ingestion of this protein in tiny amounts, but if taken in regularly they can be left feeling tired, drowsy and bloated.
Even those who do not have an intolerance should however reduce consumption, because consumption every day year in year out increases the risk of becoming intolerant.

If we have to avoid gluten, we should not only be aware of food containing this protein, such as crackers, bread sticks and rusk, but also anything with a breaded covering such as cutlets of meat or fish, fried food and even many vegetarian foods that are usually prepared with soya or wheat.
Not to forget beer, which contains malt in other words barley and certain liquors. We need to be careful with puddings, biscuits, certain types of ice cream and yoghurt and try to find gluten-free alternatives or prepare delicious dishes.

It could be trying to start with, but there are always more and more gluten-free products coming onto the market, clearly marked as such on the packaging, so you don't have to waste time at the supermarket, and once you have got the correct product in your hand things are a lot more simple.
Even if we are not gluten intolerant it is best to limit its consumption but not cut it out altogether.

# Honey and Fruit

**Fruit** can also be considered a carbohydrate as it contains fructose, which is a sugar that is naturally present in it. Fructose consumption does not cause glycemic peaks, because like all natural things it is balanced. However it is best not to exaggerate its consumption and, if we had to choose between the two we would include it with the complex carbohydrates.
On the other hand **honey** is assimilated rapidly, it has excellent properties but high quantities of fructose, so it is best not to have too much of it. It is, however, certainly better to use than sugar.

# Simple Carbohydrates

Simple carbohydrates rapidly release sugar into the blood causing sudden fluctuations of glycemia.
This results in dangerous peaks and the consequent collapses of energy, causing weakness, hunger, a longing for sugar and coffee, which in the long run causes weight gain and for whom is predisposed, diabetes.

**Sugar** is quintessentially a simple carbohydrate; it is easily and quickly digested, creating the above mentioned fluctuations.

**Bread** and **pasta**, which we regularly consume, are also derived from **white flour.**

We include in the same category **biscuits, sweets** and **sugary drinks**, that should not be consumed too often.

In addition, having lost all the valuable nutrients in the refining process, pasta is less filling and we then tend to eat a lot more of white pasta than wholemeal pasta, consequently gaining weight.

For this reason diets that avoid carbohydrates and prefer proteins are fashionable at the moment, but this is a big mistake because as we will see in the chapter on proteins, an excess of simple carbohydrates causes weight gain and in the long run problems with the liver and kidney.

As with all things one has to make compromises.

Be careful also with caffeine and tobacco; they also

cause glycemic fluctuations.

**To sum up; the refining process that foods are subjected to causes a loss in their nutritional value.**


### Challenge °2

As we have learnt, most of the food we consume is a result of a lengthy process of refinery which makes it more tasty but decreases the nutritional value, so we risk not only in failing to maintain our ideal weight, but also, even worse, developing problems with our health.

The first challenge consists of substituting, every so often, the foods which we are used to eating with wholemeal foods such as bread and pasta.

At first we might not like them, as we are accustomed to a more delicate flavour, but it is just a question of developing new habits.

So consider opting for whole wheat bread and pasta, or variants like kamut pasta or spelt, or something new we want to try. We can also try to substitute every now and again rice salad with grains of spelt, millet, oats or amaranth and experiment with new varieties and new flavours that are beneficial to our organism.

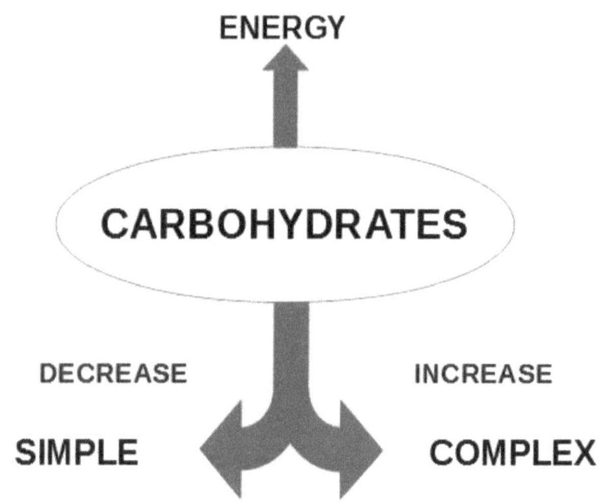


ENERGY
CARBOHYDRATES
DECREASE
INCREASE
SIMPLE
COMPLEX

# Chapter 3

Protein (what are they and what do they do?)
Protein structures
Vegetable protein
Animal protein
Today's farming
Meat
Milk
Eggs
Fish
Becoming a vegetarian
Challenge n°3

*"The extreme aversion that some adults and many children show towards meat of any type is attributed to Fitch and an atavistic tendency, namely a primitive survival instinct from our prehistoric ancestors who did not eat meat"*
**John Harvey Kellog**

# Protein

Proteins are the structural elements of living organs, meaning that they are the materials that make up cells; they are in fact composed of protein muscle and some of our organs.

Every day the proteins that we ingest are used to reconstruct our cells, produce hormones and antibodies, but, contrary to what we are used to thinking, the nutritional basic need of man is limited when it comes to protein. Protein, in fact, should make up only 10-15% of our daily food intake because it can influence our health and how we age.

The fact is, if an excess of carbohydrate is turned into fat, the protein does not get stored; whatever there is in excess gets expelled, forcing the liver and kidneys to work hard: In the long run, this tires them out and damages them, leading to illness and problems of various types.

For this reason an excessive consumption of protein is destructive, and in addition certain types of protein from animal sources are more acidic and difficult to digest.

For this reason acidification makes us more tired, with inflammation and an increase in free radicals, which are substances to be found in food that can cause various types of illnesses, early ageing and baldness (we will talk about this in our final paragraph).

It is scientifically proven that our needed daily intake is

very limited and that it is more than sufficient to take 0,75 gr of proteins for every kg of body mass; so if we weigh 75kg, our daily protein need is about 56 gr of proteins.

In conclusion, therefore, we can say that it is not the lack of proteins that is a problem but the opposite - an excess of them.

# Protein structures

Proteins are molecules made up of chains of amino acids, of which there are twenty in total. Eleven of these are not that fundamental to our body because our body produces some on its own, while the other nine are essential because we can only get them through food (two in reality are semi-essential because they are only important during our growing phase). Proteins are divided into animal protein and vegetable protein.

Animal protein contains all the essential amino acids while the vegetable ones, although containing all of the twenty, can have little or few of the essential elements.

For this reason meat has always been considered as providing a complete source of protein.

The essential amino acids present in cereals and dry fruit complement themselves with the amino acids present in pulses; therefore, their complete characteristic is calculated on the basis of our daily intake and not on a single meal. The problem, however, does not exist for vegetarians that follow a balanced diet (in addition spelt and quinoa contain all the essential amino acids and if we eat pasta and beans, for example, we would have a dish with all the amino acids required.)

Recent studies, moreover, indicate that glutenin (a protein present in cereal seeds) contains all the essential amino acids as are present in animal protein. It goes without saying that the myth of complete or incomplete protein no longer exists.

## Vegetable proteins

As we have just seen, proteins from vegetable origins present in pulses (beans, peas, chickpeas, lentils, soya, broad beans) can be considered incomplete, missing of one or more of the essential amino acids, but as we have just mentioned the magic aspect of nature is that they complete themselves with dry fruit proteins and cereals giving us a guaranteed necessary daily protein dosage.
The most difficult part to digest in pulses is their skin, the dry ones need to be soaked (between 8 to 10 hours) then cooked for a long time to make them soft and more digestible.

Adding carrots, celery, onions and alba kombu during cooking makes it all the more digestible.
Spices also come to the rescue; ginger, for example, aids digestion, while oregano and basil help to avoid feeling bloated.
**Dried fruit** and **seeds** are also a good source of proteins.
So, if we choose to follow a vegetarian diet there are fundamental foods to include in our alimentary regime.
Lentils are certainly the pulses that contain the least fat, peas provide energy and are perfect for sporty types, beans are rich in fibre, chickpeas are rich in minerals and broad beans full of antioxidants.
Soya bean on the other hand is the pulse with the highest protein value and it comes into use for a wide variety of dishes in vegetarian cooking, being in the form of milk, yoghurt, burgers and cutlets. Let's not fall into the trap of exaggeration; we must always vary our food. If we drink soya milk followed by soya yoghurt, later on a soya cutlet and finish with a soya dessert we are more or less eating the same food but in different forms.
Dried fruit such as walnut, hazel and almond contain a good quantity of vitamin E and minerals, while peanuts are high in calories.

# Animal protein

Protein of animal origin are considered superior because they contain all the essential amino acids that constitute a complete protein food while in nature these properties are scattered in various elements. Taken in small quantities alternating with vegetable protein provides us with a variety of nutritional substance which is good for our body, even if we must say that meat and fish is muscular tissue that even if lean always contains some fat.
If, however, fish has the so-called 'good' fat, for meat and dairy we are talking about saturated fat that should be consumed in moderation, and for this reason we should limit its use.
As regards their contents, animal food gives us energy but also makes us aggressive and violent, on the other hand vegetable food makes us relaxed and calm ...

# Today's farming

*"If abattoirs had walls made of glass we would all be vegetarians"*
**Linda McCartney**

Now try to imagine what the world was like hundreds of years ago.
On the small farms was a nice hen-house hosting no more than ten to twelve chickens roaming around eating grass in all tranquility with chicks by their side. Close by was an enclosure with some cows free to graze and further on up the hill a flock of sheep responding to the demands of the sheep dog.
In the enclosure behind the house a piglet was running around happily getting filthy and two rabbits chasing each other.
Now open your eyes and take a look at today's farming practices, where time is money and money counts more than people's' lives and certainly the lives of animals.
Take a look at chicken farming, where they are all enclosed in cages that at most hardly fit them, under permanent artificial lighting. They can not move and they get poorly, become aggressive and sometimes for this reason the farmer breaks their beaks.
Let's move a little further, where the chicks are checked, the females are grabbed and thrown into a

basket as we do with our washing and are used for egg production, while the males are put into machines and mashed up like we shred paper in an office because they are useless to the farmer.

In the stable we find cows that spend the whole of their lives chained up next to each other in a permanent state of pregnancy because we need milk, as soon as the calves are born they are immediately taken away from their mothers and fed with hormones to fatten them up as quickly as possible and then slaughtered after a few months and served on our tables.

Pigs, also in a permanent state of immobility, are forced to eat more than they need to.

In fish farming, fish are suffocated and left to die and in restaurants crustaceans are thrown into boiling water and cooked alive while we are unaware and smile around the table.

In addition, consider that instead of being fed with grass needed by the body, they are fed with food containing grains full of pesticides, with the addition of antibiotics to avoid disease and steroids to make them fat. These substances are partially trapped in the muscles and the result is not a happy one.

In addition fish that is not fresh is injected with bovine blood so to make the gills redder and the eye alive, frozen meat that was defrosted is sold as fresh with the further danger that when we get home we freeze it again.

Another problem are the preservative present in cold

cuts because they could become cancerogenic, as well as cheese, that only recently has been discovered to be a mixture of infected blood and normal blood.
All this phenomena leads us to be more careful about what we eat, and stops us pretending to ignore what is happening.
In the last few years some rules have started to change and some organic farming has started, where animals are free to range, living in the open air and without the use of those antibiotics and steroids, harmful not only to the animal's welfare but also to our health.
Nature provided animals to eat grass nutrients and animals that eat other animals to survive; for this reason it is not that wrong to eat animals to live on but it is mainly wrong to consider ourselves on the top of the food chain and to do as we please with other animals without the respect they deserve.
Infact, not only do we not respect them but we consequently do not respect ourselves and our health.
The main problem is that the more the years go by the more money becomes the main interest and it counts more than the health of the single person or animal.
The stock breeding of animals but also the cultivation of cereals and vegetables should be always kept under control and one should always be ever so careful.

# What can we substitute it with?

At the end of every type of food we will always find this question and the answer will contain some vegetable foods that can replace animal food for their properties.
Let's not forget that the primary substitute of animal protein are pulses.
According to some nutritionists we should not be looking for foods to substitute those of animals because they are not suitable for us and are not to be replaced, but eliminated.

# Meat

Meat is a good source of protein, but it's not as good as we are led to believe.
In fact, it contains on average only 20% protein, of which some saturated fats are added, that a result of modern day farming practices reach up to 40%, and 50% in pork.
Since the end of the war, people have started to consider meat as the only source of protein; eating meat was a sign of wealth, because the poor could not afford it and they mainly consumed their own produce from their fields.
The idea still remains that meat is the main food on

which to base a diet, but studies in the last few decades have gone the opposite way.

Up until the '80s it was advisable to eat a lot of proteins, for sportsmen, since the '90s this way of thinking has changed thanks to new research and scientific studies.

Even people that ate excessive amounts of meat had developed negative effects like cardiovascular disease and high cholesterol caused by saturated fats, meanwhile the process of meat preservation turned out to be  cancerogenic.

In the last century the increase in the consumption of meat went at the same pace of increasing health problems to the stomach and liver, and in a small way also dairy products were considered responsible.

We can therefore survive without meat and live better, but the problem apart from modern farming that greatly alters the quality not only of meat, is that there is an excessive use of it nowadays since it is served nearly with every meal.

It has therefore been established that the correct use of meat is of 1-2 times a week for white meat, while it is best to limit as much as possible the consumption of red meat.

**What can we substitute it with?**

We can find the main substitute in **seitan** a very old food that comes from Japan and has a high level of protein because it derives from wheat gluten, which as we have said is the protein of grain.

For this reason it is not good if we are gluten intolerant and also it is better not to eat it too often. On the market we also find cutlets, hamburgers, hot dogs and other products based on soya which have an excellent flavour that perfectly replaces the longing for meat.

# Milk

Like all mammals, man, from birth has a strong need for protein which is satisfied by mother's milk.
After a few months this need ceases and the first teeth appear, a sign that the baby can now start on solid food.
However us humans think that milk is needed throughout life and since we can not drink anymore human milk, we start taking dairy milk which has proteins, fats and calcium in great quantities, very useful to man.
For the above reasons it is considered a perfect food, complete and rich with many nutritious substances recommended by all.
But one needs to add that mother's milk is much sweeter and it has a lot less protein than cow's milk for the reason that us humans have different needs from the ones of a calf, that in a matter of a few weeks grows extremely fast with different requirements than a baby.

Children have also some enzymes that aid the digestion of milk that then disappear at an early age, and for this very reason adults have problems in digesting.

Two out of three people are in fact intolerant to milk without realizing it and this intolerance causes tiredness, headaches, digestive difficulties, bowel problems that up to this day we have considered normal.

On the market there are now many different varieties of milk with different effects, without lactose, etc. A clear sign this is increasingly not the kind of food for some of us.

We can also add that lactose-free milk is a highly modified milk so it is not as natural as some people say.

Milk contains calcium, but also acidic elements, and when we ingest an acidic food our body needs to transform it into alkaline which happens through calcium in bones.

Some experts claim that milk satisfies the nutritional needs only of the offspring of the mother, so mother's milk is perfect for the baby and dairy milk is perfect for the calf, but we can happily do without dairy milk.

We also have its surrogates like yogurt, a more digestible food rich in live probiotics, great to regenerate the natural flora (but not as miraculous as we are made to believe; some probiotics, in fact are inactive and useless). Another surrogate of milk is

certainly cheese, rich in saturated fats. An exception is ricotta which comes from whey and is less fatty.
So, also milk, yogurt and cheese have certain properties that can help us, while some not so much, reason why we need to think of reducing its consumption.

**What can we substitute it with?**
Nowadays it's much easier to find alternative milk products such as soya milk, oats, almond and so on, all excellent options to use for breakfast and sweets.
Instead of traditional yogurt there is soya, which can be used to make vegan cheese if we want to give it a try.
Tofu is also soya cheese, which can be used in many dishes both savoury and sweet (in its natural form it might not be so nice but with the right condiments or marinated it can be pleasant).
Yeast extract is a food enhancer that can be used to bring more flavour to pasta or soups instead of cheese.
In addition, seeds, dried fruit and certain vegetables can be richer than milk in calcium.

# Eggs

The egg is considered to be one of the most complete foods as it contains excellent sources of vitamins and minerals salts, as well as high-value proteins superior to meat and cheese. Therefore, it is transformed more easily by our body.
On the other hand it is not a good idea to take eggs if we are unwell or have problems with the liver or bowels. Apart from that it contains cholesterol (although the good one which is beneficial to us, so it is not too much of a problem).
Eggs found in big supermarkets are very often produced in intensive farms where millions of chickens live next to each other, and as we have already said, they are fed with antibiotics and chicken feed which is not ideal.
In addition, their job is to produce eggs as much as possible, so when they no longer do so, they are disposed of.
The result is the production of a great quantity of eggs of lower quality.
If we want to eat healthy eggs we need to buy organic eggs from small local farmers.

**What can we substitute it with?**
We can replace an egg omelette with a chickpea omelette, that has as many proteins and also less fats than an egg omelette.

We can also prepare some recipes using Kala-namak salt, a black salt from the Himalayas (not to be confused with the pink one, which is much easier to find) which is a salt with a sulphurous taste that resembles the flavour of eggs and is used in lots of vegan recipes.

# Fish

Fish, which is different from meat, is a type of animal whose flesh is easier to assimilate for man due to its reduced content of saturated fats.
It contains polyunsaturated fats and other important nutrients.
Macrobiotics, which means living in greatness, is a school of thought born in the east which is mainly vegan, apart from occasionally allowing every so often the consumption of fish, which is considered all right because it is healthy for our body.
Fish caught in open waters is always better than the fish-farmed fish which is artificially fed and at times with added colouring to be made look more "attractive".
There is an increasing issue that requires us to limit our consumption of fish, which is man-driven water pollution. The quantity of waste discharged by man into the sea is increasing not only in the sea but also in lakes and rivers, consequently poisonous substances

are eventually absorbed by fish.
It is always the fault of us human beings, isn't it?

**What can we substitute it with?**
As opposed to meat and dairy, there is no real adequate substitutive  elements here, because unlike meat and dairy, fish contains polyunsaturated fats which are good for us.
If we decide not to eat fish anymore we must consume a daily quantity of seeds and dried fruit, that, as we have already mentioned, are fundamental elements for vegetarians, as well as using extra virgin olive oil and seed oil.

# Becoming a vegetarian?

Studies have concluded that an excessive use of animal proteins can cause serious problems within the bowel tract, such as inflammation and tumors, while a healthy and natural diet makes us lead a better and longer life and avoids health issues in the future.
We must nevertheless take into consideration that the main problem is an excessive consumption of animal proteins, so we don't have to become vegetarians necessarily if we don't want to, but we should cut down, like it is advised in the food pyramid further on in this manual.

If we intend to become vegetarians, this is a good ethic and a healthy choice, but if our meals are based on chips, bread, pasta and refined products, sweets and various snacks, we are making a big mistake and we are running the same health risks as people who eat excessive amounts of meat.

## Challenge °3

Now that we have discovered that an excessive consumption of animal protein can be bad for us, the challenge for this second week is to start using natural alternatives.
As a change from the usual milk we try to use vegetable milk, with more pulses and less meat, we eat some soya cutlet, some tofu and seitan; in a few words we expand our boundaries.
Moreover if we are used to eating meat and meat products, a couple of weeks of rest from it, and trying to eat only vegetables can help us to detox.

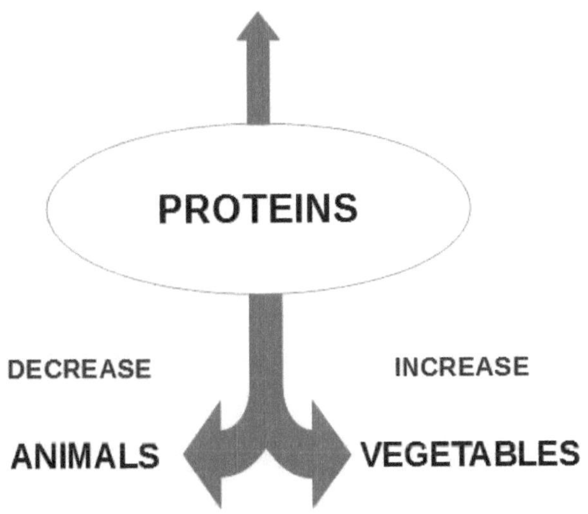
LIVE MATTER CELLS
PROTEINS
DECREASE
INCREASE
ANIMALS
VEGETABLES

# Chapter 4

**Fats (what are they and what do they do?)**
**Saturated fats**
**Unsaturated fats**
**Omega 3 and omega 6 fats**
**Hydrogenated fats**
**Challenge n°4**

*"Mass production requirements often bring with them, unfortunately, the production of the so called "junk food". The consequences are clearly visible: obesity, illnesses, early death"*

**Umberto Veronesi**
(La dieta del digiuno)

# Fats

Because of their name, they are often seen as demons and considered the main cause of weight problems and therefore the first thing we think of wanting to eliminate if we want to keep fit.
In reality, just as with carbohydrates and proteins, fats as well can be categorized into good fats, that we must take daily, and bad fats, the consumption of which we should try to limit.
The fat that our body needs reduces the risk of illnesses and diseases because it covers and protects some of our organs and our cells; fats are needed to produce hormones, they are needed to keep our skin healthy and they aid the absorption of vitamins, in addition to storing energy and strengthening the correct function of the nervous system, since 60% of our brain consists of fat.

Fats can be divided into three categories. Saturated fats, which need to be taken in moderation, unsaturated fats, which are beneficial and which should be consumed more often and hydrogenated fats, which are to be avoided as much as possible.

# Saturated fats

Saturated fats are important in small quantities for the correct functioning of the organism, but because they are to be found in small quantities in many types of food that we consume, we must try to limit as much as possible the food rich in this sort of fat, because a quantity in excess can increase our cholesterol level, increasing our weight and causing cancer  (as we have seen in animal proteins).
These types of fats are mainly to be found in **dairy food** and **meat**, especially in cold cuts and pork, but also in tropical oils like palm oil and coconut oil.

# Unsaturated fats

As with proteins, there are also fats that are essential for the very reason that our body does not produce them but gets them from food and they are the so called unsaturated fats, and these can be divided into polyunsaturated and monounsaturated fats due to their structure made of one (mono) or of more (poly) chains between various atoms.
These types of fundamental fats so important for our body are especially to be found in extra virgin olive oil (monounsaturated) but also in seed oils, seeds and dried fruit and some types of fish (polyunsaturated).

# Omega 3 and omega 6 fats

We often hear about these fats as being very important as they help tackle  problems such as depression and insomnia as well as lack of attention and they also help in keeping the heart in good health and in blood-cleansing. These fats are to be found in **blue fish**, in **tuna** and **salmon** but also in **seeds** such as linseed, sunflower, sesame, pumpkin and in the various **oils** from these seeds.

# Hydrogenated fats

These fats are not present in nature but they are chemically saturated in a way to make them less oxidized and easier to manage in many preparations, but they are not considered healthy, so they are to be completely avoided.

They are present in margarine, in some snacks, in oven-prepared products, sweet croissants and ice cream, although, in the last few years, seeing the damage that can be caused by them, they have started to become more and more replaced, but they are still present in many products (often we find them in the ingredients with the name "**vegetable margarine**").

## Challenge °4

As we have seen also fats are important in food, but in the right proportions. This week limit saturated fats from industrially produced foods as much as possible, replacing them with more beneficial unsaturated fats (instead of butter we use extra virgin olive oil on pasta and in risotto, instead of meat we try to eat fish, or if we are vegetarian we have a handful of seeds and a handful of dried fruit) we use extra virgin olive oil or oil from other seeds.

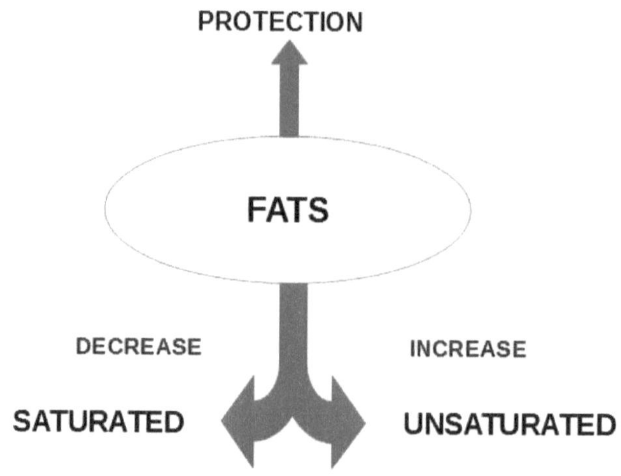

PROTECTION
FATS
DECREASE
INCREASE
SATURATED
UNSATURATED
TO AVOID: HYDROGENATED FATS

# Chapter 5

**Vitamins Minerals and Fibre**
**Fruit and vegetables**
**Chart**
**When to eat them**
**The colours of fruit and vegetables**
**Spices**
**Food supplements**
**Anti nutrients**
**Challenge n°5**

*"I am not a vegetarian because I love animals, I am a vegetarian because I hate plants"*
**Alan Whitley Brown**

# Vitamins Minerals and Fibre

Vitamins and minerals are the gears of our body, meaning that we can not produce them on our own and so we get them from food. They regulate many functions and are necessary in small quantities. Vitamins are distinguished by groups, they serve many purposes, for example they protect the skin, liver and eyes (vitamin A), they produce energy and help to correct the metabolism (group B vitamins), they create antibodies, activate enzymes and play a part in breathing (vitamin C), they introduce minerals (group D), they promote growth and stability of cells (vitamin F) and they have anti-haemorrhaging properties (vitamin K)

Minerals (calcium, iron, copper, fluoride, zinc, magnesium, potassium etc) help to combat feelings of tiredness, they participate in the correct functioning of muscles, they help bones and teeth, the nervous system, they are antibacterial, anti degenerative, and they play an important role in the production of blood cells.

So vitamins and minerals do this and many other jobs that have an important role and are not to be disregarded.

These nutrients that are fundamental to us are to be found especially in fruit and above all vegetables, which are the most simple foods, the most natural and the most healthy that our planet offers us. They cleanse us, help us to stay trim and should be consumed every day with as much variety as possible to assure that we are getting all the necessary properties from them.

As well as containing fibre, which is important for the correct functioning of the bowel and the digestive processes, vitamins and minerals are antioxidant, antiradical and are allied against ageing (not like smoking or animal fats).

# Fruit and vegetables

As regards to fruit, it must be eaten fresh and in season, because only that way it reaches the right ripeness. It contains all the nutritional values and the properties that we need in that specific moment. Infact nature gives us give the fruit we need at the right time of the year, when we have the desire for it. For example, watermelon and melon are thirst-quenching and refreshing, they grow exactly in the summer when they are most needed. Oranges and kiwis, rich in vitamin C, ripen in the autumn and winter, when we most require those substances which help us fight colds and flu.

It is rather magical if you reflect on it; it is not due to man but it is nature that delivers the right product at the right time.

In addition, if we buy fruit in season we save money, because it is cheaper as it is grown and harvested near us, reducing the cost of fuel and transport from countries far away.

An important consideration is for **exotic fruit**, which grows in very hot countries and whose properties are very thirst-quenching and refreshing.

For us living in countries with a varied and mild climate, we should avoid the above or at least limit ourselves to consume it only in the summer, because it contains vitamins and mineral salts not very useful to us in the mild season.

It is a bit as if in the summer months with a 30 degree temperature we consume a soup of hot vegetables; yes it is good for us, but in the heat we would not have the desire to eat it, we would feel even hotter and even more tired.

Exotic fruit, although to a less degree, on the contrary, refreshes our body, and therefore if we eat it in the winter we cool our body down even more and risk possible illnesses.

When we speak of exotic fruit we also include the banana, although we have come to virtually consider it as 'ours', as indeed it appears on our table all year around, as well as pineapples, mangoes, papayas and coconut.

Another reason for not consuming them is due to the long journey; they are picked unripe, and therefore not fully complete in all their substances, having failed to mature away from the tree.

So if we are lucky enough to live or go for a holiday in an exotic location, we can consume it everyday, it can be very good for us and it is much tastier than the ones found back at home because they have been picked fully mature. So let's limit ourselves to appreciate it here only in the summer.

We must not forget **algae,** that we are not used to consuming, although they do use it in the East. They are sea vegetables that feed on water and accumulate its properties, and so they contain some vitamins and minerals missing in earth vegetables, (for example vitamin B12 that is instead in meat and fish and therefore might be lacking in the diet of a vegetarian living in the west) they can also be very useful in cleansing the blood, fighting problems of being overweight, intoxication and hypothyroidism because they stimulate the thyroid gland (so it is for this reason they are not advisable for  hyperthyroidism)

# Fruit chart

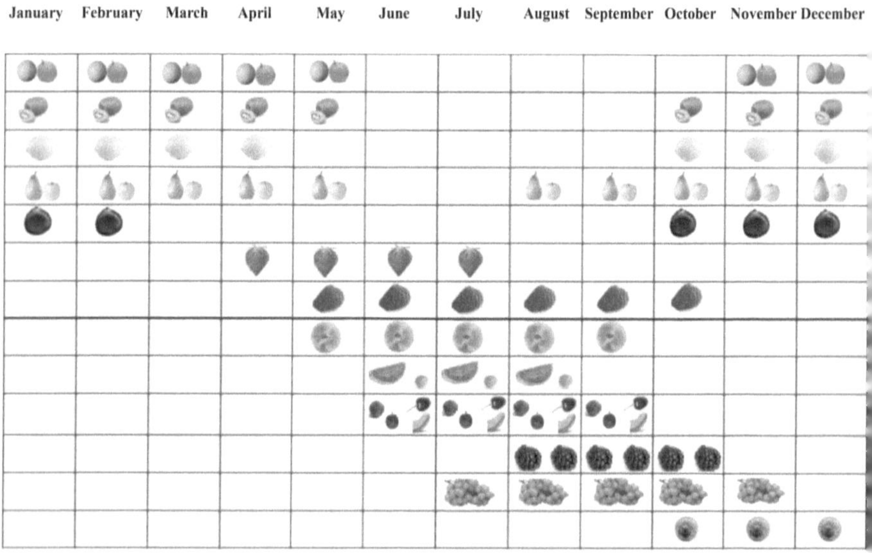

| January | February | March | April | May | June | July | August | September | October | November | December |
|---|---|---|---|---|---|---|---|---|---|---|---|

# When to eat them

# Fruit

**Oranges** and **Grapefruit**: from November to May
**Kiwis**: from October to May
**Lemons**: from October to April
**Apples** and **Pears**: all year round, apart from June and July
**Chestnuts**: from October to February
**Strawberries**: from April to July
**Raspberries**: from May to October
**Peaches**: from May to September
**Watermelons** and **Apricots**: from June to August
**Cherries, Blackcurrants, Figs, Melons** and **Plums**: from June to October
**Blackberries**: from August to October
**Grapes**: from July to November
**Persimmons**: from October to December

# Vegetables

For vegetables we can follow these general recommendations (consider that in this list some things could be defined as fruit, for example tomato and aubergine but we will call them vegetables).
**Lettuce, carrot, parsley, potato, chard, celery**: all year round.
**Artichoke, cauliflower, cabbage, fennel, leek, spinach**: all year apart from the hottest months.
**Garlic, onion, radish**: all year apart from the coldest months.
**Asparagus, peas**: spring months
**Cucumber, aubergine, sweet pepper, tomato, courgette, broad bean, rocket, beans**: between April and October
**Pumpkin**: from the end of August to the start of February

# When can they be eaten?

Fruit gets digested quickly, so it is best to eat it away from meals, such as a mid-morning break and mid-afternoon.
Vegetables on the other hand, are eaten with lunch or supper as a side dish or better, as an appetiser.
As an appetiser?
The ideal meal is to have a course at lunch or supper following a lovely salad of mixed raw vegetables, thereby rather eating raw food than something cooked. This prepares the stomach as the appetiser contains enzymes, vitamins and mineral salts which aid digestion. It also means that you eat less and so you stay trim, it gives you vital elements and eliminates toxins, reduces the feeling of a bloated stomach and strengthens the immune system.
Cooked vegetables can be combined with carbohydrates as a condiment and with protein as a side dish.

# The colours of fruit and vegetables

Another special thing about nature is represented by the colours of fruits and vegetables, of which there are five categories: white, yellow-orange, red, green and violet-blue.
They all have protective properties against the risk of tumours and cardiovascular diseases.
White: (apples, pears, garlic, cauliflower, mushrooms, onions)  the skeletal tissues, fights bad cholesterol and lowers blood pressure.
Yellow-orange: (apricots, oranges, carrots, lemons, peaches, sweet peppers, pumpkin) beneficial effect on the immune system, eyesight and keeps our skin healthy.
Red: (watermelon, cherries, tomato, radish, strawberries, redcurrants) helps memory and the urinary tract.
Green: asparagus, artichoke, lettuce, cucumbers, basil, parsley, spinach,kiwi, courgette) helps to keep bone, teeth and eyes in good shape.
Violet-blue: (aubergine, figs, blackberries, blackcurrants, plums)  helps the urinary tract and reduces the effect of ageing.

# Spices

Also spices are another gift of nature that has various benefits on our health; apart from enhancing the flavour of food they have precious nutritional elements. We can use them in abundance, for example cinnamon has disinfectant qualities, ginger, basil and oregano are digestive, clover is a tonic, cumin and nutmeg are antiseptic, sage is diuretic and anti-inflammatory.

# Food supplements

Food supplements are a weapon to help our health, but if we don't take them correctly they are useless, and can even worsen the situation.
We can use them daily to solve deficiencies, for example, as mentioned before, a vegetarian may have a deficiency of vitamin B12, but this is a vitamin that we only need in small quantities and that is stored by our body, therefore it can be useful to take a supplement of it for short periods and in cycles.
For the mentioned vitamin deficiency it is better to opt for multivitamins, because vitamins are better absorbed if in a group rather than isolated ones (the only exception being vitamin C, which is the only one we can take individually).

# Anti nutrients

Anti nutrients are those substances that damage vitamins and mineral salts, decreasing their potency and increasing our daily need of them. From this category we have tobacco, pollution, chemical substances such as medicine and pesticides, alcohol and stress.

**Challenge °5**

Let's start every day with a nice mixed salad of raw vegetables; at the start it might be a bit strange, but in the long run the positive effect will show. In addition we combine cooked vegetables to our first and second courses, creating the right nutritional balance made up by a salad, followed by a first or a second course with the inclusion of cooked vegetables.

INDISPENSABLE TO
STAY HEALTHY
VITAMINS & MINERALS
FRUIT
VEGETABLES

# Chapter 6

**Food combinations**
**Carbohydrates and protein**
**Protein and protein**
**Carbohydrates and carbohydrates**
**Flour and yeast**
**Pulses and cereals**
**Eggs, meat and fish**
**Dairy**
**Vegetables**
**Fruit**
**Jam and cereals**
**Challenge n°6**

*"Make food your medicine and medicine your food"*
**Hippocrates di Coo**

# Food combinations

It is not just important what we eat, but also what we eat with it.

Incorrectly combining food provokes the same defects that are caused when we eat unhealthy food, such as a prolonged period of digestion that makes our digestive system work unnecessarily hard, a sense of tiredness and lethargy and an incomplete breakdown of food.

Food that is assimilated rapidly such as carbohydrate should not stay too long in the stomach, whereas proteins need enzymes, gastric juices and time to break down. Carbohydrates need an alkaline environment while proteins, on the contrary, an acidic one, that is why it is advisable to always eat a first course for lunch and a second course for supper, or the other way round.

**Protein with protein** is a combination to absolutely avoid (so meat, fish, dairies, eggs and pulses must be consumed on their own and not combined with each other) as all proteins have different structures and require long and different digestive processes.

Also **carbohydrate with carbohydrate** is a combination to avoid, although more tolerable.

So we can break the rule sometimes but not always.

## Flour and yeast

It is important to moderate the intake of leavened products, like for example bread, pizza, crackers, bread-sticks, dried biscuits etc, because they have a gluey effect on our intestinal tract, caused by the yeast and the gluten, making digesting long and difficult.

## Pulses and cereals

The combination between these two nutrients (see the famous pasta and beans) creates a complete combination where in one dish all the essential amino acids are found.

On this combination there also different views, some nutritional experts disagree because of the excess of starch.

It is up to the individual to try and see the effects after this combination (two parts cereal/one part pulse)

## Eggs,meat and fish

Eggs, meat and fish are best combined with vegetables.

If we cannot avoid bread we can still eat it but without exaggerating.

Likewise for a nice glass of wine with meat and fish.

## Dairy

With cheese, bread is ok.

As it is for milk to be put in cornflakes.

It is better to avoid coffee and milk because caffeine makes the digestion of milk more difficult.

We can substitute normal coffee with barley.

**Vegetables and vegetables**
Vegetables go perfectly well with each other and are well combined with protein and various carbohydrates, (with the only exception of fruit that is best eaten alone).
Vegetables are very good as an appetiser or side dish, such as salad, cauliflower, mushrooms, courgettes, asparagus, artichoke, rocket, carrot or anything you fancy, following recipe or using one's imagination.
The only vegetables to watch out for and limit (do not consume every day) are from family solanaceae, e.g. **potato, aubergine, tomato, pepper**, because they are acidic foods and contain solanine which is toxic to the liver if used daily.
Tomatoes are very acidic and best associated with proteins; pasta with tomato sauce is not the best combination, but it is ok if not eaten everyday.
This is the same for potatoes that go ok with meat and eggs occasionally but not too often.

**Fruit**
Fruit is best eaten alone, away from meals, because it works better to detox and reintegrate minerals.
Eaten as a snack, at tea time or in the morning, fruit contains fructose, a sugar that is easy to digest and that goes right through the bowel giving us energy; but if the bowel is already full of food previously eaten and being digested, the fruit stays stagnant, waiting for

the previous food to be digested, and in the meantime fermentation sets in. This causes further weight on digestion, creating discomfort, stomach ache and when finally digested a lot of the valuable properties in fruit has been lost.

In general, apples and pineapple for their properties are the fruits that can accompany meals every so often.

Fruit also do not go greatly with vegetables, with the exception of some energy or detoxing juice that we can prepare at home (the same goes for milk, in the form of an occasional milkshake).

## Jam and cereals

Rusk biscuits and jam have always been considered a perfect pair, but some disagree with the association between jam or honey (simple sugars) and cereals, like rusk or bread, so best to eat jam alone.

We can conclude that vegetables are the best to use as side dishes, maybe we are accustomed to a little green salad and nothing more but the world of vegetables offers hundreds of types of food. All we need is a bit of curiosity and our side dish is served.

## Challenge °6

In this paragraph let's start following food combination rules correctly and let's eat in the right order, as shown in this chapter.

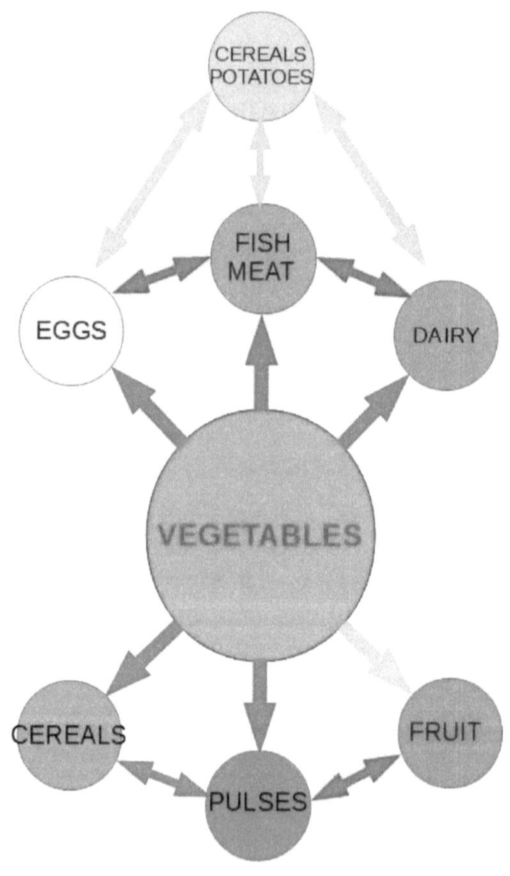
CEREALS
POTATOES
FISH
MEAT
EGGS
DAIRY
VEGETABLES
CEREALS
FRUIT
PULSES

# Chapter 7

**Preservation of Food**
**Fresh produce**
**Frozen produce**
**Dry produce**
**Packaged and vacuum packed**
**Fermentation**
**Mistakes in preservation**
**Challenge n°7**

*"We, the consumers, buy the product created by an industry obsessed with profit without complaint, thereby contributing the finance of this disaster"*
**T Colin Campbell**
[Whole, vegetable and brown]

# Preservation of Food

Eating **fresh produce** is the best way to feed
ourselves. They contain all the properties and quality
and are at the best nutritionally. If, however these
products come from far away it means that they have
been picked when not fully mature, so it is best to
choose fresh organic produce from zero km, or better
still, our own produce, if possible.

**Frozen produce** has its advantages in that it is frozen
as soon as it matures, and so does not need additives
or preservatives added to it, as long as the process has
been correctly followed, so the product keeps all its
properties intact.

Whenever possible it is best to cook it from frozen as
the with the defrosting of the product water is lost,
and with it, the nutritional value such as vitamins and
enzymes. Food left to defrost also gives bacteria a
chance to alter the product which can be an important
problem.

**Dry produce** such as pulses need to be soaked to get
rid of toxins that may have developed during the
drying process. It is also important to thoroughly cook
these products to avoid potential intestinal problems.
Using these tricks we can consume food rich in
properties without the losses that occur during
defrosting.

Certain grain cereals may also need a soak; on the pack
it says if it does need it or not, and for how long,

however more than often it is not necessary as before packaging the grains are usually precooked or toasted, making soaking unnecessary and easier to eat if all we are left to do is cook them.

The use of **canned and vacuum packed food** is to be reduced because it has lost most of its nutritional values and contains a lot of salt or preservatives that altered its potency.

The process of **fermentation** causes the formation of micro-organisms that help the bacterial flora; sauerkraut, yogurt, vinegar and oriental food like tempeh, miso, tamari and shoyu are produced in the oriental culture and extracted by fermenting soya.

# Mistakes in preservation

All food contains bacteria that when frozen go into a state of sleep; when it is defrosted they come back to life and start to multiply. If we freeze it again, we freeze a food with a high level of bacteria, that once defrosted again will multiply once more contaminating even more the food with the risk of becoming toxic. However, if we cook food for the first time and then freeze it, the bacteria is less and is killed off during the cooking process.

## Challenge °7

Avoid tinned or frozen food and try go more often to the greengrocer and to cook fresh food and in season.

# Chapter 8

**Cooking food**
**Raw**
**Steamed**
**Stewed**
**Grill**
**Oven**
**Microwave**
**Fried**
**Challenge °8**

*"When the last tree is cut down and the last river is poisoned and the last fish is caught, only then will we realize that we cannot eat money".*
**Native American Indian proverb**

# Cooking

It is fundamental for nutritional value how we cook food; some foods must be cooked to be safe because heat kills germs, but others, like fruit and vegetables, is better to consume raw because heat reduces or eliminates all the vitamins and mineral salts, altering their composition.

It is as important to vary cooking style as it is having a varied diet.

Ovens and pressure cookers generate a lot of heat and have a warming effect, ideal in the cold months; we can use the griddle or the gas for steaming, but **raw** food is more refreshing and keeps much better its nutritional value.

The less cooking we impose on food the more vitamins and minerals remain unadulterated; this is especially true with fruit and vegetables, which are better to be eaten as they are. So, let's eat raw, as much as possible.

**Steamed** cooking is a way of cooking that maintains nutrients more like what they are in nature and it is better used for vegetables and fish.

Stewing also keeps the elements in good condition, and it is great with fish.

The **griddle** is very versatile, we can just quickly warm up vegetables or fish and meat.

The **oven** is great for meat and fish but without roasting too often because that type of cooking causes the formation of free radicals.

**Microwave** cooking has divided the sceptics, some consider it damaging while others think it is safe.

The problem is that scientists are confused on the effects of this sort of cooking.

However, it is certain that electromagnetic waves are released which modify essential fats. So avoid cooking fatty food, like fish and meat.

We could use the microwave sometimes for quick dishes.

It is clearly known by everyone that **fried** food should be limited as much as possible because it is the least healthy method of cooking a food due to the long contact in hot oil that makes the food less nutritionally valid and more dangerous for our health.

This is because fried food (like all food which is burnt or roasted) develops free radicals which attack and destroy the good fat in our body, increasing the future risk of contracting illnesses.

For this reason one should not eat fried food more than once a month (or try even less).


**Challenge °8**


For this week consume more raw food and less cooked food, no fried or roasted food. In addition, by differentiating the style of cooking, but also the type of vegetables cooked, we will have both a different and a pleasurable taste.

# Chapter 9
## The food pyramid challenge n 9

*"Nowadays millions of people don't have access to drinking water, yet to produce one kilogram of beef 20.000 litres of water is needed"*
**Umberto Veronesi**
(The fasting diet)

*"A carnivore diet is greatly responsible for famine that is still afflicting many populations of the countries in the so-called developing world"*
**Margherita Hack**
(Why I am a vegetarian)

# Food pyramid

The food pyramid was invented to give an idea on how to base a correct diet.
The lower part of the pyramid shows food that needs to be consumed in great quantities everyday; the more one goes up to the top the more the food should be limited.
We will find below two pyramids that show a healthy diet, a mix between a Mediterranean pyramid and the oriental on the right side, and an optimal diet, the vegetarian one, on the left.
Then we will find a list of all the food to consume each day, on alternate days, occasionally or rarely.

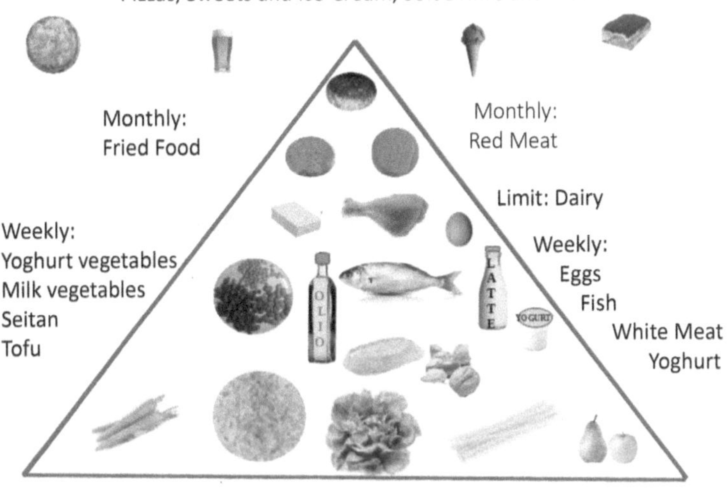


Everyday :
Wholemeal cereals
Vegetables
Fruit

Everyday with
moderation:
Oil
Pulses
Dried Fruit

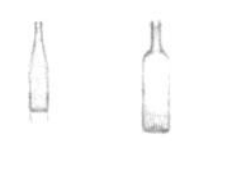

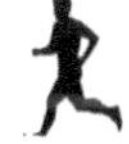

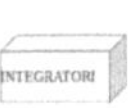


Drinks one or two
litres of water
everyday

Physical exercise
daily

Food supplements

**Challenge °9**

Now that we are familiar with the food pyramid, we can decide on what to base our diet on and to use the rule of the 80% -20%; this means that we try to follow for 80% of the time the correct diet and we could afford a 20% of "concessions" (for example a pizza at the weekend, or a slice of cake on another day or some culinary treat).
Now that all the challenges have ended we move on to the summary and to the last details to get to know more in depth our food.

# Chapter 10

**Food Guide**
**Every day**
**In small quantity**
**2-3 times a week**
**1-2 times a week**
**Occasionally**
**Rarely**

*" To eat correctly not only prevents illnesses but it generates good health and a feeling of well being"*
**T.Colin Campbell**
(The China Study)

# Food guide

We find below a list that sums up the many nutrients and advice for their usage.

## EVERY DAY

### Vegetables
Vegetables should appear in large quantities on our table, both at lunch and supper, raw and cooked.
To be consumed every day.
With the exception of tomatoes, potatoes, aubergines and peppers; these are not to be eaten every day.

### Fruit
Fruit should be eaten  every day, especially between meals, in a snack or before breakfast, it should be in season so that all nutritional properties are present.
To be consumed every day.

### Cereals
As we have already seen there are a lot of cereals and ideally they should be consumed every day, and varied, avoiding repetition. Whether it is grain, rice, spelt, oats, amaranth, quinoa, millet, maize, barley or rye, the important thing is to vary them so to get all the nutrients and the characteristics that each cereal possesses.
To be consumed every day.

## Pulses

If we are vegetarian we can eat a small quantity of pulses as a main protein meal every day or alternated with the animal protein.

## Seeds and dried fruit

Seeds and dried fruit are especially important for vegetarians (but also for meat eaters) although they should be eaten in small quantities.

## Oils

Choose cold-pressed oil because hot-pressed oil, while generating more oil, losses all its properties.

Extra virgin olive oil is extracted from the first cold pressing of the fruit, while the simple olive oil from is heated pressing of the remaining fruit and comes from processes of refinement which renders it nutritionally poorer.

So extra virgin olive oil goes well on everything, everyday while simple olive oil is ok once in awhile.

Other oils (of linseed, maize, sunflower, sesame, peanut and cod liver oil) contain excellent qualities and complement olive oil, we can use them daily or in turn, adding extra virgin olive oil to give extra quality to our dish.

On the other hand, tropical oils are not recommended due to the high content of saturated fats.

Soya oil is an industrially produced oil and therefore should be avoided or taken very rarely.

## Green tea, herbal drinks and barley coffee

Green tea can be taken daily because it healthy and protective, but not the bottled version that has sugar and additives.

Herbal drinks and infusions, especially before bedtime, can be used regularly.

Feel free to drink barley coffee, much better for you than normal coffee.

## N.B. Curative foods

Fruit and vegetables are protective foods that fight against illnesses and disease, but I want to make two things plain.

Firstly, **lemon** is a magic fruit on which many books have been written praising its thousands of properties; it is acidic to the taste, but it is not at all acidic for our body, on the contrary, it has an alkaline effect and it helps to prevent acidity. We can, for example use the juice to dress salads or drink it with a bit of tepid water in the morning as soon as we wake up.

Secondly, **garlic** is a medicinal food, it is also a natural antibiotic due to its properties that are beneficial to the whole body.

## TO LIMIT

### Vinegar

Most industrially produced vinegar contains sugars and flavouring so the best choice is to use cider vinegar that has beneficial qualities for digestion and limit all other types of vinegar such as balsamic vinegar.

### Salt

Salt should be used parsimoniously as it increases blood pressure. Best to opt for wholegrain salt. When we are preparing pasta it is best to dissolve it in the cooking water and not to put it directly onto the pasta.

Best to substitute salt with gomashio, which is sold in supermarkets. We can also make it up ourselves and save money; all you need is sesame seeds which have been washed and toasted in a pan and sea salt crushed in with it. One part salt to between seven to twelve parts sesame seed. This way our food is tasty but has the addition of the qualities of sesame, with less salt.

### Sugar

White sugar is not a nourishment, it has empty calories that make us fat but do not feed us. We can use it to sweeten our drinks but in small quantities. If we are used to having a lot of sugar in our drinks, we should try to cut it down slowly and get used to something less sugary, then we will realise that we like food that is not as sweet as we were used to having.

Raw cane sugar is much better, better still honey or malt (coming from barley it therefore contains gluten), leaves of stevia (a herbaceous plant and a potent sweetener).

Maple syrup, agave nectar, soaked and blended dates that create a natural and sweet paste are all perfect to make sweets and puddings.

## Milk and yoghurt

Changing the type of milk every week is a good method, so is using almond milk, oats milk, hazel, soya and rice milk.

Even if we want to use dairy milk, it is advisable to alternate it with vegetable milk.

The same goes with yoghurt, which we consume daily, but it is not as necessary as the media makes out.

## Chewing gum

Even if we do not swallow it the sugars and the substances present are absorbed by our saliva so it is best not to consume too much of it and avoid chewing gum with sugar.

## Caffeine

Caffeine creates dependency; those who drink it do not feel any better than those who do not drink it, but they feel better before drinking it due to a psychological and habit-created routine. Caffeine is in tea as well, but has a milder and prolonged effect. Coffee wakes you up quickly, but soon after one has the urge to have more, while there is not the same effect with tea, but it lasts longer.

Caffeine is a toxic substance produced by some plants, in a sort of defensive action and it has a stimulating and exciting effect, but it is not good for us, especially if used more than once a day.

## Parmesan cheese

As with all cheese, parmesan contains fat, but we can use it daily in small quantities. We can substitute it with yeast extract.

## 2-3 TIMES A WEEK

## Fish

Fish contains polyunsaturated fats and other excellent qualities that make it the animal food to eat it more often.

We are talking about blue fish such as sardine, mackerel, herring and anchovies, but also fish such as cod and salmon go well if we rotate them. As for prawns and clams, we can have them occasionally. Remember that freshly caught seafood is always better than farmed fish and frozen fish.

**Bread and polenta, bready snacks and crackers**
Bread is all right if accompanied by main meals but it is better to restrict it, even if we are used to eating it. Alternate polenta with other types of bread or grain crackers.

## 1-2 TIMES A WEEK

### Meat
White meat such as chicken or turkey contains less fat and so can be eaten once a week.

### Eggs
The egg is a complete food with more easily digested protein than meat or cheese, but it should be consumed in moderation seeing it is already present in lots of foods such as pasta, sweet products and biscuits.

### Cheese
Cheese contains protein but also lots of saturated fats and salt (even mozzarella), so best to choose organic and local cheeses.

## OCCASIONALLY

### Pizza

Best made at home when possible, with less fat and salt than in a restaurant or from a takeaway.

### Chocolate

Milk chocolate while being an anti-depressant, it contains too much sugar and saturated fat. Not advisable.

Dark chocolate containing 70% cocoa or more has anti-cancer properties and antioxidants, so we can take it more often, also in the form of bitter chocolate or powder (an excellent alternative being carob chocolate which comes from a tree to be found around the Mediterranean).

### Ice-cream

Homemade ice-cream is better as it contains less fat than industrial ice-cream, so we can consume a bit in the summer as it is so refreshing and makes us feel better.

### Refined snacks

Snacks made from refined ingredients contain fats and sugars and so are best if taken only occasionally.

### Biscuits

The same goes for biscuits, however biscuits provide calories and so are ok from time to time, maybe at breakfast.

## Home made cakes and biscuits

These could be a suitable alternative at breakfast or as a snack as they are light and may not contain milk and eggs which would make them a lot more fatty.

## Stock cubes

These contain a lot of salt, the better ones are vegetarian. When possible it is better to prepare a homemade broth, although we could use a stock cube every now and then, but try to use a stock cube that does not contain fat, or substitute it with **miso**, a fermented product from soya and barley or rice, to add at the end of cooking to flavour soups and very rich in proteins, microbiotic and enzymes.

## RARELY

## Cakes and sweet snacks (and fizzy drinks)

Most of the sweets that we find on the market contain a high quantities of sugar and fat, so it is better to take them only on special occasions.

## Sweets and toffees

Apart from ruining teeth, they are very bad for us due to the high content of sugar and artificial ingredients. Take them as little as possible.

**Ketchup and mayonnaise**
Much better if home-made, they do have a lot of fat.

**Butter and margarine**
Butter has saturated fat and cholesterol, while margarine is based on vegetables, but it does not exist in nature and has a lot of hydrogenated fat. It is better to choose butter, although even better to avoid both.

**Cold cuts, red meat and fried food**
Cold cuts and red meat have a high quantity of saturated fat. In addition cold cuts contain preservatives that are cancerogenic.
Fried food, apart from the loss in nutritional value, causes the production of dangerous substances like free radicals.

**Alcohol, tobacco**
The only exception is red wine that sometimes we can take with meals in small quantities. As regards to other types of alcohol it is better to cut them down to a minimum because they not only cause liver problems but they increase blood sugar levels, just like it happens with refined food, the same with tobacco that causes problems to lungs and throat.
In addition they cause early ageing. Some expert consider alcohol, tobacco and meat to be a form of slow poison, because their excessive use in the long run will make us feel bad.

# Chapter 11

**Organic and chemical products
Organic?
What to watch out for?**

*" Food, one assumes, gives us nutrition; but
Americans eat it fully aware that small quantities of
poison have been added to improve its looks and to
delay rotting"*
**John Cage**

# Organic?

The word organic started in opposition to the damage caused by additives, pesticides, pollution and chemical changes that are used more and more by farmers to produce better harvests at minimum cost.
To be classified as 'organic', vegetables can not be cultivated in fields where specific rules are not respected, for example if fertilizers and pesticides are used.
The use of preservatives and colouring are not allowed, as well as pesticides, sprays and chemical fertilizers.
In addition, organic fields must be a good distance from the ones that use chemicals and they must be kept natural for at least two years before being considered organic.
If animal farming is to be classified 'organic' the landowner must respect certain rules, like in the abuse of hormones and type of food fed to the animals, maintaining a clear difference between intensive farming where the end result is really not healthy.
It is true that in any case we are never really totally sure of how our food is produced, so the best thing is to have a small vegetable patch at home. If this is not possible it is better to choose organic food, and so making sure we bring to our table as little poison as possible.

# What should we watch out for?

Genetically Modified (GM) foods are food products that have been modified with genetic engineering techniques and the result is a type of food that is not natural and potentially risky to health and the environment.

To keep food fresh additives and preservatives are useful; but there are contrasting views regarding the risks to our health.

They are innocuous in small quantities, but there are always more and more foods with them, so we must be careful. The same goes for colouring and flavouring agents, derived from petrol, emulsifiers, solvents, thickeners, sugar substitutes, flavour enhancers and many more chemical products, every single one with a use. It is good to remember to eat mainly natural food, without too many ingredients and manipulations. This is the most correct and right thing to do.

# Chapter 12
**Use and Instructions**
**Breakfast**
**Snacks**
**Lunch**
**Dinner**

*"There are things that have to be done every day; eating seven apples on a Sunday night instead of one every day simply will not have the same effect"*
**Jim Rohn**

# Breakfast

Many people say breakfast is the most important meal of the day, but in spite of this it is the most underestimated.
Breakfast should be the most complete meal and include carbohydrates (cereals, fruit or honey) proteins and polyunsaturated fatty acids (dried fruit, seeds or ideally vegetable yoghurt), vitamins, minerals and fibre (always in the form of fruit or cereals).

Ideally, we should drink first thing in the morning a glass of tepid water with lemon juice, which as we have seen is a fruit of a thousand proprieties, or a freshly made fruit juice (not from a carton) of oranges, kiwis, pears, apples, blueberries; some type of fruit that is in season. Also let's try to vary it as much as possible, because each fruit has its own cleansing and regenerating effect and we assimilate the proprieties best of all in the morning, on an empty stomach.

After a quarter of an hour we can start our balanced breakfast which consists of cereals like muesli, with some vegetable milk, adding a handful of seeds (sunflower, linseed) and dried fruit (almonds, pine kernels, walnuts, hazelnuts, not so often peanuts as it is the most fatty of all dried fruit).
On sale we can find oats muesli with seeds and dried

fruit, or just oat flakes.

A good solution to those who don't like seeds or dried fruit is to blend it and to put it in a sealed container and add milk, so we take in all their properties without realising, and if we are not that keen on muesli, we can just add our favourite cereal.

If we like it and it makes us feel good we can have jam and pitta bread, which is unleavened bread and more easily digested than normal bread.

Fruit, that is always better to be taken away from mealtimes, can always be eaten before breakfast (as juice) or mid-morning and the meal is complete.

If we don't like eating too much at breakfast time, we can have a fruit salad.

## Snacks

Mid-morning and afternoon snacks are the most important.

Suggestions for quick snack according to preference:

-one or two fruit or a fresh fruit salad without sugar (every day if possible vary the fruit according to what is in season)

-home made fruit juice (not ready prepared as it contains water, sugar, flavouring and very little real fruit)

-a handful of dried fruit

-one yoghurt

-one natural yoghurt with a cup of berries

-cereal cakes
-crackers
-biscuits
-snacks

# Lunch

We can choose a lunch based on complex carbohydrates to ensure we get the right amount of energy needed throughout the day and choose a meal based on proteins that requires a prolonged digestion and relaxes us in preparation for our night's sleep (try to eat at least three hours before going to bed).
Raw and cooked vegetable should never be missing. Let's start our meal with a healthy mixed salad, and then move onto our plate of wholemeal or cereal seed pasta, together with some sauce prepared with cooked vegetables, or with small portions of animal protein.

# Supper

As with lunch, vegetables should not be missed out, then we can have a protein food varying between vegetables or animal, and occasionally accompanied with wholemeal bread or polenta, but at least three hours before bed.

Instead if we work nights, we can choose a supper based on carbohydrates to avoid feeling heavy by the long digestion time and have protein for lunch.

Also in this occasion have a mixed salad, a protein food, a side dish of cooked vegetables or cereals like bread.

Supper should be the lightest of the three meals; to avoid problems at night we should eat less (nightmares and insomnia are also related to what we eat just before going to bed), as opposed to what we usually do, because we tend to have a fast breakfast, we eat a fast lunch and only in the evening after a rushed day at work we give ourselves the pleasure of a meal sitting at the table.

# Chapter 13
## Basic rules

*" For a healthy life the only rule is moderation. This means moderation in all healthy things"*
**Herbert MacGolfin Shelton**

# Basic rules

Remember to chew food well and to give yourself enough time during a meal, avoid using if possible TV, smartphone, newspapers and too difficult conversation.

Changing a diet can make us feel worse in the first few days, this is because our body is used to a certain lifestyle and to suddenly change it (I am not talking of small improvements, but a total change) at first can put us out and make us decide to go back to our old way.

This is a problem that might only take a few days for us to adapt.

If we modify our diet gradually, changing something every week, we would not have any problems.

Food routine is very important , if we want to regulate our well being we must try to get up, have lunch, dinner and go to sleep possibly always at the same time.

A lunch based on carbohydrates is easy to digest and gives us energy for the rest of the day, while a meal based on protein requires a long digestion time, so it must be consumed for supper, at least three hours before going to sleep.

If we ate protein for lunch we would feel more tired than usual in the early afternoon due to the long

digestion process that they cause.
Carbohydrates give us the energy and the strength to face the day, while protein rebuild the cells.

We can use the 80%-20% rule for food, so if our diet is 80% healthy, we can afford to break rules from time to time, like one meal a week or one or two days a month of food not exactly healthy. This does not represent a big problem, instead it is mentally healthy to break rules from time to time, rather than becoming slaves of nutrition and other regimes.
Natural food is curative and protective unlike a meat diet, therefore if we increase the consumption of meat we are more exposed to diseases.
We must choose wholemeal food that preserves all the nutritional qualities, and especially avoid fried or burnt food and refined and manipulated food that contains artificial additives.
Our body is alkaline, the very opposite of proteins which are acidic, especially the ones from animal origins, so when we eat an acidic food our body must work very hard to get back to normality; this is why proteins from animal source are only good in small quantities.
Let's conclude by saying that the maximum level of healthy efficiency for a balanced diet is reached when we eliminate smoking and stress and we increase physical exercise.

# Part 2

**Vegetarian Recipes**
**What to have in the house?**
**Quick and easy recipes**

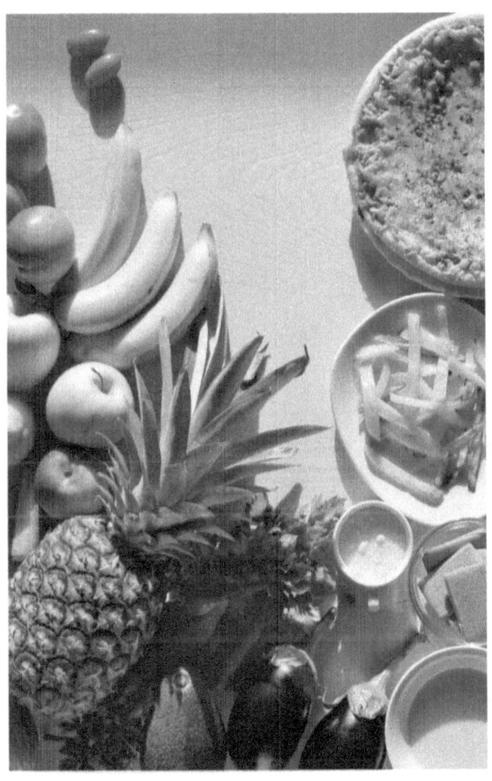

# What to have in the house?

**A short list of what we might need if we decide to turn vegetarian.**

## In the fridge
vegetable yoghurt
vegetable milk
varied seasonal fruits
varied seasonal vegetables
tofu
seitan
tahini (sesame sauce)

## In the freezer
frozen vegetables
frozen fruit (for desserts)
cutlets, hamburgers and other soya preparations

## In the larder
dried fruit and seeds
cereals for breakfast
pasta and various cereals
dry pulses

algae
tinned food
various flours
yeast
sodium bicarbonate
various spices
maize starch
cocoa (or carob flour)
biscuits without milk or eggs
coconut flour
dates
maple syrup or agave nectar

## At hand

extra virgin olive oil
seed oil
brown sugar
whole grain sea salt
cider vinegar

## Recipes

Here is a small collection of quick and easy recipes to prepare, some gluten free, others with raw food, but all of them vegan, tasty and good, for breakfast, lunch and dinner, with appetisers and condiments.

# BREAKFAST

## Almond milk

**Ingredients:**
a cup of almonds
three cups of water
a handful of de-stoned dates

**Preparation**
in a container leave the almonds to soak overnight.
-Dry and blend them together with three cups of
water, a handful of dates (dates will make the milk
sweet, add a few at the time and taste them until the
right sweetness is reached).
-Drain with a small mesh strainer
-Your milk is ready


Instead of almonds you can use other types of dry
fruit, for example hazelnuts, or coconut flour to make
coconut milk.
The almond paste left in the strainer can be used for
other recepies, for example to prepare a seed cake with
avocado cream or to make biscuits.

# Assorted muesli

**Ingredients:**
one cup of sun flour or walnut oil
one packet of oat flakes
one packet of crunchy muesli
as much as you want of dry fruit (blueberries, bananas, raisins), dark chocolate flakes (as you prefer)
-To start with grind the seeds with the walnuts
-Mix all the other ingredients together in an airtight container and eat it gradually every morning.

# Seed cake and avocado cream

**Ingredients:**
for the base
250gr sunflower or linseed oil
almond milk paste (as you want)
3-4 dates

for the cream
one soya yoghurt
two mature avocados
one glass of soya milk
one tablespoon of cocoa
one and a half of brown sugar
coconut flour to sprinkle

-Mix all the ingredients of the base together
-Lay them on a plate
-Blend together the cream ingredients (if the mix is too thick add a little soya milk)
-Spread the the cream on top of the base
-Decorate with grated coconut and keep in the fridge.

# Tea-time biscuits

**Ingredients:**

250gr of spelt flour (or plain flour)
half a glass of vegetable milk
one spoon of almond milk paste (or in alternative grated coconut)
one tablespoon of seed oil
one tablespoon of brown sugar
one teaspoon of sodium bicarbonate
cinnamon, cocoa (if you wish)

-Combine flour, sugar, oil, bicarbonate and the almond paste (or coconut) and start to mix adding the vegetable milk a little at the time.
-Lay the mix and flatten it with a rolling pin and with shapes make the biscuits.
-Bake at 180°C for 15-20 minutes.

# Carob cream

**Ingredients:**
200gr peeled hazelnuts
100gr brown sugar
carob flour
one tablespoon of peanut or sesame oil
vegetable milk (as needed)
Here is a simple and fast recipe to prepare a delicious cream, to consume also in the morning with pitta bread.
The quantity of carob flour is left for us to decide, so is the milk to add to reach the desired consistency.
-We can add raw hazelnuts or toast them in the oven or on the pan for a few minutes, to make the cream last longer.
-Add the sugar and oil to the ground hazelnuts.
-Add the carob flour, the vegetable milk a little at the time, so to create a creamy consistency.

# Fruit shakes or fruit salads

Another good way to start the day is by drinking a blend of fruit with mixed vegetables, here we can use our imagination and mix anything we fancy, or with a fruit salad with no more than three fruits, to avoid digestive problems.
We can also prepare a green smoothie, made by blending green leaf vegetables (with even more beneficial properties) with celery, spinach, cucumber or courgettes, basil and parsley, with varied fresh fruit to assemble a mix of vitamins and excellent nutritional properties like with apple, lemon and pear.

Also we can opt for the classic style mixing oranges, carrots, and lemon or a kiwi and melon for a cleansing and refreshing juice.
Pineapple and lime, with a sprinkle of coconut flour for a tropical taste, or peaches, strawberries and a piece of watermelon for a summery taste.

# LUNCH

## Spelt Pasta

**Ingredients:**
350gr spelt flour
125-150 ml of water
salt
extra virgin olive oil, spices, tomato sauce (to taste)

Preparing home-made pasta is very simple and very quick.
Here is a recipe with spelt flour, but we can prepare it with other types of flour following the same instructions.
-In a bowl mix flour, a pinch of salt and add water little at the time and work by hand for 5 to 10 minutes to create a firm dough.
-Lay the dough with a rolling pin to the required thickness and cut the pasta to make long strips to make fettuccine (if we improve we can make without problems ravioli or tortellini shapes and with a pasta machine make spaghetti etc.)
-Cooks in few minutes
-We can add to the dough olive oil, tomato paste, spices, or anything we like to give the pasta more flavour or a different colour.

# Barley with pumpkin

**Ingredients:**
200gr of barley
vegetable stock
pumpkin pulp
one onion
extra virgin olive oil

-Fry the onion, add the pumpkin pulp cut into small pieces and into the hot stock and leave to cook for 5-10 minutes, until the pulp is soft.
-Squash the pulp with a fork, add the barley and carry on cooking until the barley is cooked.

# Potato Gnocchi

**Ingredients:**
500gr of potatoes
100gr of wholemeal flour (or flour of other cereals)
salt and oil

-Boil the potatoes with their skins on until soft.
-Once cooked peel them under running water so not to burn and squash them.
-Add salt, sieve the flour and work for a few minutes into a firm dough.

-Now take a piece of dough and form some strips and cut them into gnocchi.
-Cook in boiling water for a few minutes.

# Soya Spaghetti

**Ingredients:**
250gr soya spaghetti
one onion
one courgette
80gr of mushrooms
80gr of soya bean sprouts
soy sauce

-Cut carrots and the courgette Julienne style, and the other vegetables into squares.
-In a pan fry the onion, add the carrots, courgette, mushrooms and soya bean sprouts.
-Drop the soya spaghetti into boiling water and cook for two minutes, then drain, add the soy sauce and toss them a couple of times with the vegetables.

# Rice with vegetables

**Ingredients:**
250gr of rice
500ml vegetable stock
one onion
half a glass of white wine
a little saffron
100gr of mushrooms
100 gr of green beans
five cherry tomatoes

-Warm up the vegetable stock, in the meantime gently fry the onion.
-Steam the green beans, slightly cook the mushrooms then put them aside.
-Add the rice and let it toast for a few minutes.
-Add the white wine, and when completely evaporated add some vegetable stock and cover all the rice until it starts to evaporate.
-Towards the end add the saffron , the vegetable mix and serve.

# Risotto of 5 cereals

**Ingredients:**
250gr of 5 cereals (ready packed at the supermarket,
with spelt, barley, rice, kamut and oats)
one onion
oil
two large courgettes grilled Julienne style
a pinch of yeast extract
salt
500ml of vegetable stock
chopped parsley

-As for risotto with vegetables warm up the vegetable
stock, in the meantime gently fry the onion.
-Add the cereals to the onion and toss for one minute,
add a little stock and cover.
-Carry on mixing and adding stock and a pinch of
yeast.
-Towards the end add the courgettes, a little oil and
mix.
-Turn off the heat, add the parsley, mix and serve.

# Spaghetti with tofu

**Ingredients:**
200gr wholemeal spaghetti
200gr soya bean sprouts
3 tablespoons of soy sauce
a packet of tofu
one onion
chillies
extra virgin olive oil

-Cook the spaghetti.
-In the meantime in a pan soften the onion, the tofu (previously cut into small squares and dried) and the soya bean sprouts all for a few minutes.
-Add to the drained spaghetti, the soy sauce and toss for a few minutes.

# Couscous

**Ingredients:**
couscous
two leeks
a courgette
a carrot
mushrooms
soy sauce
250ml water

-Cut the carrots Julienne style, toss courgettes and leeks in the pan.
-Bring water to the boil with a drop of oil and a pinch of salt, in the meantime put the couscous in a bowl and pour enough water to cover it completely.
-Put a top on the cereal bowl and let it rest (follow the instructions on the packet)
-Put the couscous in the pan with the vegetables, add the soy sauce and mix for a few minutes.

# Millet burger

**Ingredients:**
200gr of millet
one aubergine
one courgette
one potato
2 tablespoons of of bread crumbs
a pinch of cumin
oil
salt and chillies

-Cook the millet, in the meantime cut the potatoes into small pieces and grill the potato, the courgette and the aubergine.
-As soon as the millet is cooked add it to the grilled vegetables.
-Add the cumin and breadcrumbs a little at the time, until hard (the quantity of breadcrumb varies depending on the type of millet used)
-Once cooled down shape the burgers and put into the oven at 180°C for 15-20 minutes.

# Quinoa and Amaranth Quiche

**Ingredients:**
150 gr of amaranth
150gr of quinoa
spinach
garlic
oil
salt and pepper
breadcrumbs (as you like)

-Wash and cook both the amaranth and quinoa.
-Steam the spinach and then toss them in a pan with
the garlic and oil.
-Make two layers of amaranth, and quinoa and spinach
in the middle.
-Cook in the oven at 180°C for 10-15 minutes.

# GARNISHES AND CONDIMENTS

## Pitta bread

**Ingredients:**
300gr of flour (gluten free; wholemeal, spelt)
about 150ml of water
a drop of extra virgin olive oil
a pinch of salt

-In a bowl put together flour, oil, salt and the water a little at a time, mix into an homogeneous consistency.
-Leave to rest for half an hour under a towel.
-Divide the paste into small balls and flatten them with a rolling pin to form round discs.
-You can cook it in the oven at 180°C for 15 minutes, or toss it in a pan for a few minutes on each side.
-We now have a very light and easily digestible bread to eat for breakfast with jam, carob cream or as a garnish to your meals.

# Mushrooms

**Ingredients:**
one tablespoon of maize oil
300gr of clean and cut mushrooms
pepper
the juice of half a lemon
garlic and parsley (as you like)

-Wash and cut the mushrooms into strips, in the meantime warm up the pan with the maize oil, pour the mushrooms on top and mix.
-Add pepper a little at a time, the lemon juice, if you wish the garlic and parsley, and mix until the mushrooms are cooked.

# Guacamole

**Ingredients:**
one ripened avocado
one onion
a lime (or a lemon)
salt and pepper to taste
one tomato, olives, chillies (as you like)

-Guacamole sauce is a very old recipe from the Aztech period, originally made with avocado, lime and salt.
-In a bowl mix the avocado in small pieces with the lime juice, squash it with a fork to make it creamy.
-Add an onion (and if you wish tomato, olives or chillies) cut into small slices, salt and peeper and leave to cool in the fridge for a few hours.

# Crispy Baked Potatoes

**Ingredients:**
four large potatoes
extra virgin olive oil
salt

-Peel the potatoes, cut them as you wish an leave them in water for half an hour so they lose their starch.
-In the meantime preheat the oven to 220°C.

-Drain and dry the potatoes, cut them into slices, and put in the oven with a sprinkle of oil and salt for 25-30 minutes at 180°C.

# Hummus

**Ingredients:**
200gr of chickpeas
1 tablespoon of tahini (sesame cream)
a clove of garlic finely chopped
the juice of one lemon
fresh parsley
a sprinkle of oil
salt and pepper

-If you are using dried chickpeas, leave them to soak overnight, drain and steam for an hour before using them.
-Instead if you use tinned ones, you can put all the above ingredients in a mixer until a creamy consistency is reached.

# Pea puree

**Ingredients:**
200gr of peas
some basil leaves
salt
pepper
vegetable stock

-Cook the peas and the basil in the vegetable stock for 10 minutes.
-Put the peas, a bit of stock, salt and pepper and blend.

# Yoghurt spinach

**Ingredients:**
300gr of spinach
70gr of soya yoghurt
one leek (or onion)
one tomato
the juice of half a lemon
salt
oil
-Steam the spinach, in the meantime fry the leek (or the onion), add the chopped tomato, lemon and salt and cook for a further 5 minutes.
-Add the spinach and cook for another 5 minutes.
-At the end of cooking add the yoghurt and mix, salt to taste and serve.

# SUPPER

## Vegetable stock

**Ingredients:**
one onion
two carrots
celery
a clove of garlic

-Chop all the ingredients and fry with some extra virgin olive oil.
Now we can use it for cooking as it is, or add more ingredients like fennel, tomato, spices for example oregano, basil and ginger, or seaweed.

Add pulses like beans and peas to make delicious minestrone or soups.

# Pizza

**Ingredients:**
200gr of gluten free flour
180ml of water
15gr of yeast
a pinch of salt

for the wholemeal flour:
if we want to create a dough with wholemeal flour we have to mix 100gr of plain flour with 100gr of wholemeal flour for a crispy result.

For the mozzarella cheese:
50gr of natural soya yoghurt
50 ml of soya milk
30gr of maize starch
a pinch of salt
a touch of maize oil
mix everything into a liquid cream

Add to the flour water, yeast, a drop of oil and a pinch of salt then work for a few minutes to create a soft dough.
-Now leave it under a cloth to rise for about three hours.
-Prepare the mozzarella adding all the ingredients in a bowl and mix well to a liquid but creamy result.
-When the dough has risen, lay it and roll it out into

the desired thickness; brush on the tomato sauce, pour drops of mozzarella cream and all the other ingredients that we wish to use and bake in the oven at 200°C for 10/15 minutes.

# Pumpkin flower burgers

**Ingredients:**
15 pumpkin flowers washed and cut into small pieces, pistil removed
200 gr gluten free flour
100-150ml of water (depending on the type of flour)
one teaspoon of bicarbonate
salt

-Prepare the batter by adding the flour, bicarbonate and salt and warm water little at the time.
-Stir with a whisk creating a sort of creamy effect rather than a dough
-Put the pumpkin flowers in the batter and mix well
-Put them in a hot frying pan with some oil (we do not need to use oil if it is a non stick pan), spread the cream all around the pan  and cook on a slow flame for a few minutes on each side.

# Seitan with lemon

**Ingredients:**
200gr of seitan
for the marinade
two tablespoons of soy sauce
two tablespoons of extra virgin olive oil
a sprig of parsley
lemon juice
a small slice of ginger root
one teaspoon of maize starch
150ml of water
salt

-Start to marinade by mixing together the soy sauce,
oil, lemon juice, ginger and finely chopped parsley
-Cut the seitan into small slices and leave it to marinate
for over an hour.
-Cook the seitan on a griddle for a few minutes on
both sides.
-Meanwhile melt the maize starch in the lemon juice
and add water.
-When the seitan is cooked, lay it on a plate, pour the
liquid just prepared into the pan until it thickness.
-Turn the gas off and pour it over the seitan.

# Aubergines with tofu

**Ingredients:**
a block of tofu
two aubergines
garlic
extra virgin olive oil
tomato
oregano

-Wash and cut in a half lengthways the aubergines, let them drain, cover with sea salt, cover with a plate and let the liquid drip for one hour, this is useful to eliminate the bitterness in the aubergine.
-After this, put the aubergines in boiling water and let them boil for a few minutes, then drain again.
-Now hollow the aubergines with a spoon and remove the inside pulp completely, to make a sort of shell to put the filling in.
-In a pan prepare the filling by frying the squashed garlic with a little oil.
-At this point cut the tofu and the remaining aubergine into small cubes and with the tomato sauce and the oregano pour into the pan.
-Leave it to cook for a few minutes until the aubergines are perfectly cooked, add the necessary salt, remove from the heat and put the filling aside.
-Fill the aubergine shell with the prepared sauce, cook in the oven for 20 minutes at 180°C.

# Tofu on toast

**Ingredients:**
a block of tofu
sliced bread
extra virgin olive oil
oregano
tomato sauce
salt

-Toast the sliced bread in the oven or in a pan.
-In a pan heat the chopped tofu, add the tomato sauce,
the oregano, salt,  and ingredients as you wish
(mushrooms, artichokes, olives) and cook a few
minutes.
-Rub a clove of garlic on top of every slice of bread
Add the extra virgin olive oil, the tofu sauce and serve.

# Asparagus and chickpea omelette

**Ingredients:**
150gr chickpea flour (gram flour)
100gr boiled asparagus cut into pieces
300gr of water
one leek
a little seed oil
salt and pepper
spices (to taste)

-In a pan gently fry the leek and the boiled asparagus cut into small squares.
-Mean while prepare the batter mixing water and the chickpea flour, add some salt, pepper and spices as you wish to form a thick cream.
-Pour the cream evenly into the pan with the leek and the asparagus and after a few minutes lower the flame and let it cook for 6-8 minutes.
-Turn the omelette and cook the other side too so to create a slight crispy crust.

# Beans in sauce

**Ingredients:**
200gr beans
50gr of tomato sauce
one onion
a clove of garlic
parsley
salt and pepper

-Cook the beans until soft (if the beans are dry leave them to soak in water overnight) and add salt at the end.
-Fry the garlic and onion, add tomato sauce and pepper.
-Blend half the beans with the tomato sauce and a little cooking water, and pour into the plate, add the beans as a whole, the minced parsley and serve.

# Peas in guacamole

**Ingredients:**
400gr peas (frozen or fresh)
guacamole sauce
sliced rye bread

-Prepare the guacamole sauce
steam the peas for 8-10 minutes
-Mix the peas with the guacamole sauce
-Toast the bread and serve it with the sauce.

# Stewed Lentils

**Ingredients:**
200gr lentils
one potato
vegetable stock
oil
bay leaf
onions
wine

-After having gently fried the onion and potato add
the lentils deglaze with wine.
-Add the vegetable stock and the sliced tomato and
leave it to cook for 40 minutes, until the lentils are
ready.

# SWEETS & DESSERTS

## Soya pudding

**Ingredients:**
500ml soya milk (at room temperature)
3 spoons of maize starch
3 spoons of agave syrup (or 2 of brown sugar)
cocoa (for the chocolate version)
vanilla (for the vanilla version)
cloves (or anise)
cinnamon

-In a pan mix together milk and the maize starch until
the starch is melted.
-Put the pan on the flame.
-Add the agave syrup (or the brown sugar), vanilla, (or
cocoa if you fancy a chocolate one) and some cloves.
-When it is close to boiling and starts to thicken
remove with a spoon the cloves, keep mixing, pour
into bowls and sprinkle with grated cinnamon.

# Pudding cake

**Ingredients:**
500gr vanilla soya pudding
500gr cocoa soya pudding
dry biscuits without milk or eggs
cinnamon (or cocoa)

-Prepare in two separate pans the pudding (see above).
-In a plate for sweets, form a base for the dry biscuits, pour over the warm vanilla pudding, then make another dry biscuit layer and pour over the cocoa pudding.
-Carry on with the layers of biscuits, vanilla e cocoa pudding.
-Sprinkle with cinnamon (or cocoa)

# Broken biscuit cake

**Ingredients:**
200gm dark chocolate
200gr of biscuits
50gr vegetable oil
50gr seed oil
dates

-Melt the chocolate in a double boiler, in the meantime brake the dry biscuits in a mixer together with the dates (previously soaked overnight) milk and oil.
-Spread the mixture on the greaseproof paper, pour the melted chocolate and shape as a small salami.
-In the fridge a few hours and it is ready.
We can also use black cocoa instead of dark chocolate.

# Mango cake

**Ingredients:**
for the base
300gr dry biscuits without milk or eggs
2 tablespoons of brown sugar
vegetable milk

500gr of soya mango yoghurt
200ml of vegetable cream
6 tablespoons of vegetable milk
15g natural gelling agent (agar agar)
cocoa (to sprinkle)

-Chop in a mixer the dry biscuits, add sugar and a little vegetable milk just to make the paste wet.
-With the paste make the base and leave it in the fridge for half an hour.
-Prepare the cream by adding to the yoghurt the whipped vegetable cream and lay the paste over the base.
-Again in the fridge for over an hour.

# Chocolate sponge

**Ingredients:**
200gr flour
100gr of maize starch
two tablespoons of cocoa
three tablespoons of sugar
half a sachet of baking powder (or a spoon of
bicarbonate)
one tablespoon of oil
200ml vegetable milk

-In a bowl mix all the ingredients a little at a time.
-Mix for a few minutes to create a solid dough.
-Put in the oven for half an hour at 180°C

# Coconut and cocoa truffles

**Ingredients:**
dates
coconut flour
cocoa
mint (as you like)

-In a mixer blend all the ingredients and create a homogeneous  and solid mix to be able to shape little balls to put in the fridge and serve cold.
-For every 10 dates we add about half a tablespoon of coconut flour and half of cocoa, plus two mint leaves.
-We can also make sweets just  with cocoa or just with coconut, and others with mint to add colour to our dish.

# Bibliography

AA.VV., 2011, Il libro completo dei rimedi naturali, Giunti Demetra

AA.VV., 1998, Curarsi con il cibo, La Biblioteca Ideale Tascabile

AA.VV., 1998, Le diete che funzionano, La Biblioteca Ideale Tascabile

Aspre Barbara, 2008, Il tuo cibo dalla A alla Z, Tecniche Nuove

Berioni, Calvi, Croci, Melgiovanni, Zugnoni, 1987 Errori alimentari, a tavola senza veleni, De Vecchi Editore

Buonfino Liliana, 1977, La cucina integrale, Mondadori

Casati Elio, 1993, Il grande libro della cucina vegetariana, Mariotti

Carr Allen, 2008, È facile controllare il peso se sai come farlo, Ewi Editrice

Campbell T. Colin, 2005, The China Study

Campbell T. Colin, 2013, Whole, Vegetale e Integrale, Whole Rethinking the Science of Nutrition, Macro edizioni

Carper Jean, 1998, La giovinezza vien mangiando, Sperling & Kupfer Editore

Chaitow Leon, 1999, La dieta della lunga vita, Edizioni Red

Ciaburri G., 1974, Cucina Vegetariana, salute e longevità, Sperling & Kupfer

D'Elia Armando, Guidi Antonella, 2012, Miti e realtà dell'alimentazione umana, Si Edizioni

Dalla Via Gudrun, 2007, La dieta dello sportivo, Edizioni Red

Dalla Via Gudrun, 2008, Le combinazioni alimentari, Edizioni Red

Del Vantesimo Ada, 1990, La dieta italiana, Sperling Paperback

Djokovic Novak, 2013, Il punto vincente (Serve to win), Sperling & Kupfer

Formenti Alessandro, 2007, Mazzi Cristina, La salute in cucina, Edizioni l'Informatore Agrario

Granger Laura, 1991, Calcio e alimentazione, Ulisse Edizioni

Hack Margherita, 2011, Perché sono vegetariana, Edizioni dell'altana

Hittleman Richard, edizione aggiornata 1993, Yoga, esercizi, concentrazione, alimentazione, Mondadori

Holford Patrick, 2009, La salute comincia a tavola, Vallardi Editore

Kousmine Catherine, 2004, La tavola della salute, Giunti

Maffei Franca, 1999, Guida alle combinazioni alimentari, Demetra srl

Maugeri Paola, 2012, La mia vita a impatto zero, Mondadori

Menassé Iginia, 1981, La conservazione di frutta e verdura e la congelazione di tutti gli alimenti, De Vecchi Editore

Momentè Stefano, 2007, Cargnello Sara, Solo crudo, Macro Edizioni

Mozzi Piero, 2012, La dieta del dottor Mozzi, Mogliazze

Pedrotti Walter, 1997, Il cucchiaio verde, come curarsi con il cibo, Demetra

Pellati Renzo, 1994, Alimentazione per la famiglia, Fabbri Editore

Rifkin Jeremy, 1992, Ecocidio, Mondadori

Strozzi Silvia, 2011, Cereali che bontà, Macro Edizioni

Todisco Mauro, 1994, La cronodieta, Tecniche Nuove

Veronesi Umberto, 2013, La dieta del digiuno, Mondadori

## Courses

Audio-corso di Alimentazione e salute, Trevisani Catia, 2011, Edizioni Enea
Corso conoscere il cibo, Ermes srl
Corso dimagrire con l'alimentazione, Ermes srl

## Web sites

Iltuocorso.it, per i corsi online
Frasicelebri.it, per le frasi e citazioni
Benessere360.com
My-personaltrainer.it
Nutrizionenaturale.it
Focus.it
Universobio.com
Vegfacile.info
Veganitalia.com
Giallozafferano.it

**Cristian Ortlie** is an expert, passionate about food and ways of improving well being through yoga and meditation.
After many different professions in different fields he now focuses on writing simple, practical manuals that help to change our lives.
Contact: cristian.ortile@gmail.com